Sleep Apnea

The Ultimate Guide on Diagnosing and Treating Sleep Apnea

The Alternative Healing Series

Hayden Anderson

Copyright Act of 1976, the scanning, uploading and electronic sharing of any part of this book without the explicit written consent or permission of the publisher constitutes unlawful piracy and the theft of intellectual property.

If you would like to use material or content from this book (other than for review purposes), prior written permission must be obtained from the publisher.

You can contact the publishing company at admin@speedypublishing.com. Thank you for not infringing on the author's rights.

Speedy Publishing LLC (c) 2014
40 E. Main St., #1156
Newark, DE 19711
www.speedypublishing.co

Ordering Information:
Quantity sales; Special discounts are available on quantity purchases by corporations, associations, and others. For details, contact the "Special Sales Department" at the address above.

This is a reprint book.

Manufactured in the United States of America

Table of Contents

Publisher's Notes i

Chapter 1: Introduction 1

Chapter 2: Three Types of Sleep Apnea 4

Chapter 3: The Signs and Symptoms of Sleep Apnea 7

Chapter 4: How Sleep Apnea is Diagnosed 10

Chapter 5: Diagnosing Sleep Apnea with Sleep Studies 15

Chapter 6: Sleep Apnea Symptoms in Children 19

Chapter 7: Treating Sleep Apnea 22

Chapter 8: Making Lifestyle Changes 24

Chapter 9: Other Treatments for Sleep Apnea 26

Chapter 10: Important Facts About Sleep Apnea 36

Chapter 11: Conclusion 38

Meet the Author 39

More Books by Hayden Anderson 41

Publisher's Notes

Disclaimer

This publication is intended to provide helpful and informative material. It is not intended to diagnose, treat, cure, or prevent any health problem or condition, nor is intended to replace the advice of a physician. No action should be taken solely on the contents of this book. Always consult your physician or qualified health-care professional on any matters regarding your health and before adopting any suggestions in this book or drawing inferences from it.

The author and publisher specifically disclaim all responsibility for any liability, loss or risk, personal or otherwise, which is incurred as a consequence, directly or indirectly, from the use or application of any contents of this book.

Any and all product names referenced within this book are the trademarks of their respective owners. None of these owners have sponsored, authorized, endorsed, or approved this book.

Always read all information provided by the manufacturers' product labels before using their products. The author and publisher are not responsible for claims made by manufacturers.

Print Edition 2014

Chapter 1: Introduction

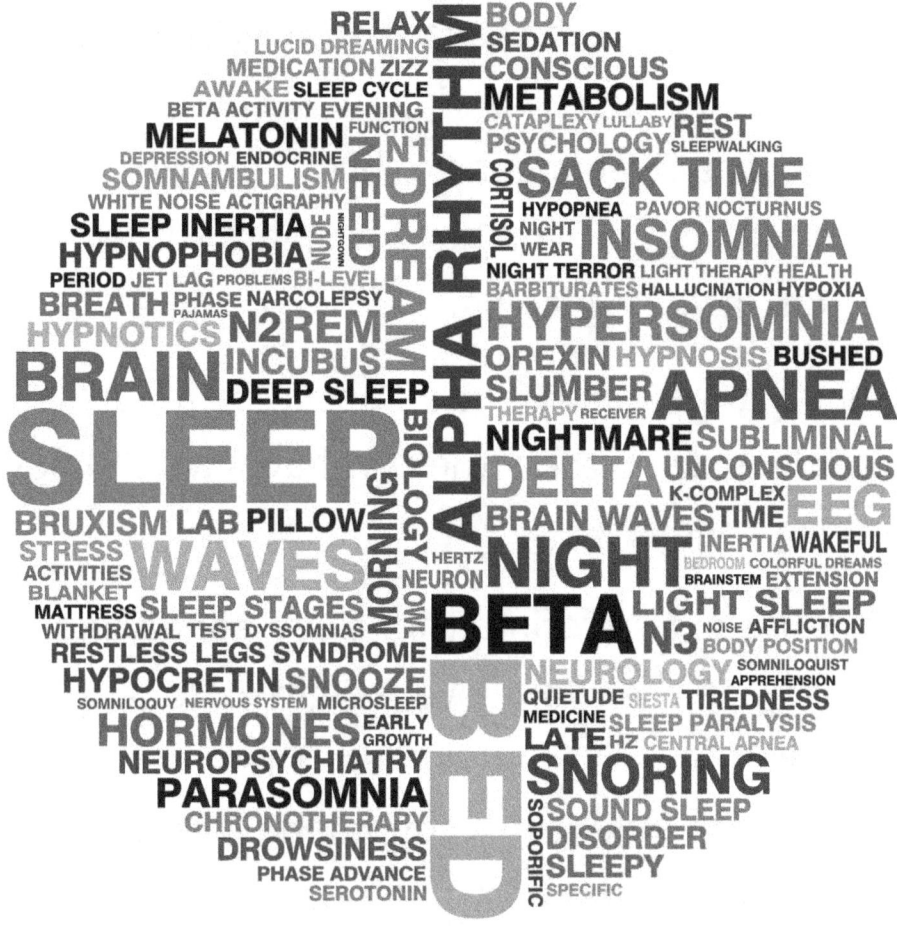

Sleep apnea is a condition when you temporarily stop breathing while you're sleeping or the breaths that you take are shallow. The temporary breathing can last from a few seconds and go on for a few minutes. These breathing interruptions can happen so many times an hour, even more than thirty times within a sixty minute time span.

Afterwards, you will breathe normal again. It may be accompanied by loud snorting or choking. This condition can interrupt you from getting a good night's sleep. It causes you not to get as much sleep as you need to. Sleep apnea causes you to be tired and sleepy during the day.

This condition is not one of those that are easily diagnosed. Also it is usually not detected during a regular exam with your physician. Because it happens while you are sleeping, you probably don't know that you have it unless someone notices an unusual pattern in your sleeping.

The way that you may find is if a spouse or a partner notices it while you're sleep. Even then, they probably won't know that you may have sleep apnea.

Millions of adults are suffering from sleep apnea and don't know it. The majority of them are overweight or obese. Men suffer from this condition more than women. The older a person is, the more likely they can inherit this condition. With women, they can develop sleep apnea in the post-menopausal stage of their life.

More minority groups, such as African-Americans, Hispanics and Pacific Islanders develop sleep apnea more than other ethnic groups. It can also be inherited from a family member. If you have small airways in your throat, mouth or nose, you are more likely to have this condition.

Young children that have larger than normal tonsil tissues can also develop sleep apnea. You can also be at risk for sleep apnea if you:

- Smoke
- Have high blood pressure
- At risk for having a stroke
- Heart Failure

CHAPTER 2: THREE TYPES OF SLEEP APNEA

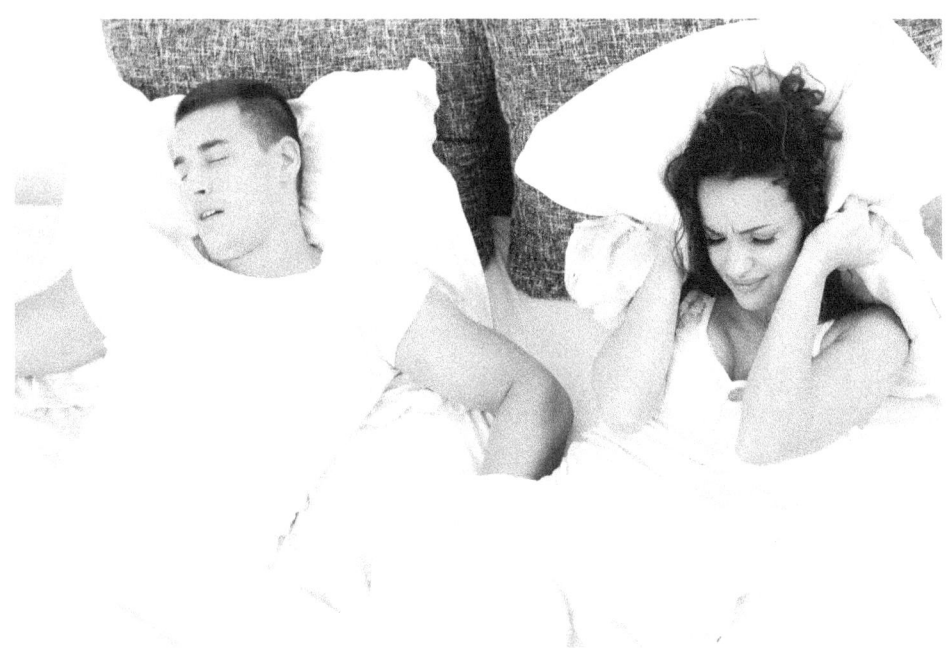

There are three types of sleep apnea, however only two are discussed the most. There is obstructive sleep apnea, which is the most common type for this condition. With obstructive sleep apnea, your throat muscles collapse while you're sleeping.

The other type of sleep apnea is called central sleep apnea. This type happens when your breathing muscles do not receive the right signals. The third one, which most people don't experience, is called complex or mixed sleep apnea. This type is a combination of both conditions.

Obstructive Sleep Apnea

Obstructive sleep apnea, or OSA, blocks the air passage in your throat. Some other things that happen with this type of sleep disorder are:

- While you're sleeping, the throat muscles collapse inward as you're breathing.

- Air will go through the upper airway. This includes the nose, mouth and throat areas.

- As the muscles get wider, they block the collapse in order for the airway to remain open.

- You will have less oxygen in your blood. This causes your lungs to absorb air from the outside.

- Apnea happens when the back throat tissues are temporarily blocked. You stop breathing and if you wake up you may have to gasp for breath.

- Even if you do gasp for air or make snorting sounds, you may not necessarily wake up.

If you experience five or more apnea episodes per hour, it is considered to be part of obstructive sleep apnea.

Central Sleep Apnea

Central sleep apnea is not as common as obstructive sleep apnea. This type of sleep apnea starts in the brain (central nervous system). The brain will not send a signal to the airway muscles so that they can breathe.

The level of oxygen decreases and you will probably wake up. With this type of sleep apnea, people usually remember waking up. If you have heart disease or heart failure, then you are experiencing central sleep apnea.

Complex or Mixed Apnea

As mentioned earlier in this report, this is the combination of obstructive and central sleep apnea. With this type of sleep apnea, you will deal with obstructive sleep apnea, or OSA. In addition to that with good pressure from the airway, you will also have central sleep apnea.

If you are using CPAP (Continuous Positive Airway Pressure), the central sleep apnea will be acknowledged. This happens after the obstruction has been cleared.

Chapter 3: The Signs and Symptoms of Sleep Apnea

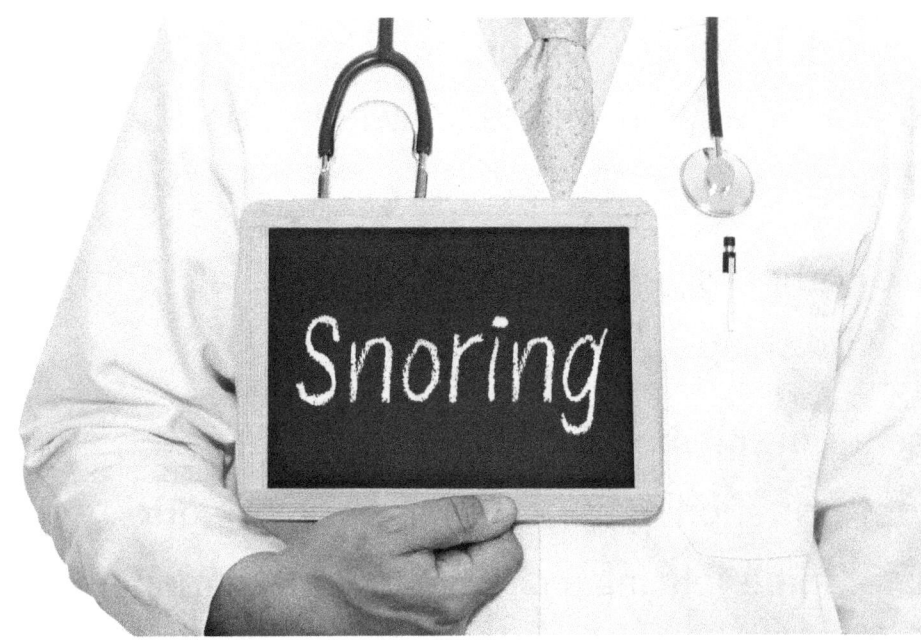

The most obvious sign of sleep apnea is snoring that is loud and consistent. You may pause while you are snoring. You may also choke or gasp after you have paused. When you sleep on your back, the snoring gets louder. If you sleep on your side, the snoring may not be as loud.

You may or may not snore every night. Eventually, the snoring may increase and it may get louder as you sleep.

Since you're sleep while you're snoring or gasping, you may not know that you're having breathing issues. Others will see the signs before you and will let you know if it becomes a pattern. Be aware that just because you may be a chronic snorer, it doesn't mean that you have sleep apnea.

If you are fighting sleep during the day, that could be a sign that you have sleep apnea. If you're not engaged in any activity, you may end up falling asleep very quickly. If this happens while you're at work or you're driving, the chances are greater that you may end up in a work-related accident or an accident while you're driving.

There are other signs and symptoms that people may not associate with sleep apnea. They are:

- Headaches in the morning
- Frequent urination in the evening or night hours
- Moody or experiencing a change in your personality
- Can't concentrate, focus or loss of memory
- Dry throat in the morning as you wake up

The muscles in your throat are used to keep the airway open so that you can get air into your lungs. However, when you're sleeping, your throat muscles are relaxed. This means that your airway can be blocked and air won't get into your lungs.

With obstructive sleep apnea, you can also experience the following:

- If you have a tiny structure at the head and neck, the size of the airway may be smaller in your mouth and throat.
- The muscles in your throat and your tongue are more relaxed than they should be.

- Being overweight or obese, you will have additional soft fat tissue. This tissue can get thick in the windpipe wall. There is not much of an opening and what is available may not stay open.
- If you are an older adult, the signals of your brain may not keep the muscles of your throat stiff like they should.
- With the blocked airways, you may end up snoring loudly as you sleep.

Low oxygen levels cause you not to be able to get a good night's sleep. The muscles in the upper airway get tight and your windpipe is open. You are able to breathe normal again, until you start snorting or choking.

Along with the frequent low levels of oxygen and less hours of sleep, your stress hormones are released. This can cause you to have high blood pressure, a stroke, heart attack and abnormal heartbeats. The stress hormones can also cause you to have heart failure.

If your condition is not treated, you could be at a greater risk of obesity and diabetes.

CHAPTER 4: HOW SLEEP APNEA IS DIAGNOSED

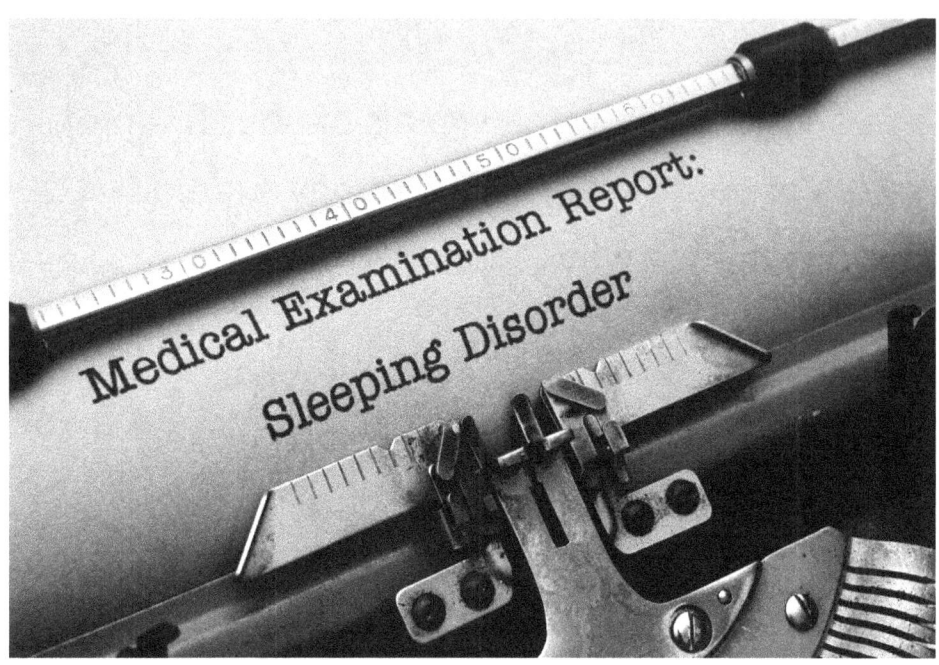

The way that physicians diagnose sleep apnea hinges on medical and family histories. They will also conduct a physical examination. They will study your symptoms. If they feel that the signs, symptoms and patterns fit this condition, then you will be referred for a sleep study.

Sleep studies are measurements that show your sleeping pattern. The results show how much and how well you sleep. If you have any problems with your sleeping, the studies will show the results of that.

If you are referred for a sleep study, it is important that you get one. The study can determine if you have been diagnosed with a sleep disorder, such as sleep apnea. Sleep apnea and other sleep disorders can increase your health risk for strokes, high blood pressure and heart attacks.

Physicians who are experienced in reading sleep studies can easily diagnose sleep apnea and provide treatment so that you can sleep better at night. The important thing is to let your physician know about any adverse sleeping habits you have experienced.

They would include fatigue and chronic sleepiness during the day. Also, advise your physician if you've had difficulty getting to sleep or waking up in the middle of the night and can't go back to sleep.

You could be suffering from a sleep disorder that you are unaware of. Physicians experienced in sleep disorders will ask you about your sleep schedule. They will also ask your family members about any chronic snoring that they have dealt with.

Physicians who are experienced with sleep disorders are known as sleep specialists. They can easily diagnose and provide treatment for those who are experiencing problems sleeping.

In order to help the specialists pinpoint what's going on, you should create and keep a sleep diary for no more than two weeks. This is the prelude to the sleep study. Here are some questions that you may see on a sleep diary:

- The time you went to bed the previous night
- The time you woke up in the morning
- How many hours you slept the previous night

- How many times you woke up during the night
- How long did it take you to fall asleep the previous night
- What medications you took the previous night
- If you were you wide awake when you woke up in the morning
- If you were you awake and tired when you woke up in the morning
- If you were you sleepy when you woke up in the morning
- The number of drinks with caffeine did you have during the day
- The number of alcoholic drinks did you have during the day
- The time that you consumed the alcoholic drinks
- The number of naps you had
- How long the naps lasted
- If you were very sleepy during the day
- If you were a little tired during the day
- If you were somewhat alert during the day
- If you were you wide awake during the day

Your physician may also inquire with you to ask the following:

- Snorting
- Gasping
- Headaches in the morning

If the results of the diary determine:

- Frequent naps
- Wake up more than a few times during the night
- Takes you more than a half hour to get to sleep

- Constantly sleepy in the daytime

Physical Exams to Check for Sleep Apnea

During the physical exam, your physician will check the areas of your throat, nose and mouth. They will be looking for enlarge or additional tissues. For children who are diagnosed with sleep apnea, they usually have enlarged tonsils. With them, it doesn't take much to provide a diagnosis other than an exam and medical history.

For adults, the physicians look for an enlarged uvula, which is a piece of tissue that sits and hangs from the middle of the back of your mouth. They also look for a soft palate, which is in the back of your throat and is known as the roof of your mouth in that area.

How Family Members Can Help to Detect Sleep Apnea

Because most people don't know that they're suffering from sleep apnea, it's important that there is someone that can detect abnormalities while you sleep. The person doesn't know that their breathing can start and stop at any time during the night. They also don't take into consideration when someone tells them that they are a chronic and loud snorer.

There are things that family members can do to help out:

- Let them know that they have a chronic case of loud snoring.
- Ask them to consult their physician.

- If they are diagnosed with sleep apnea, advise them to follow the instructions, including any post-op follow up and treatments.
- Be there for them emotionally. This can be a trying time for them, and they need all of the support that they can get.

Chapter 5: Diagnosing Sleep Apnea with Sleep Studies

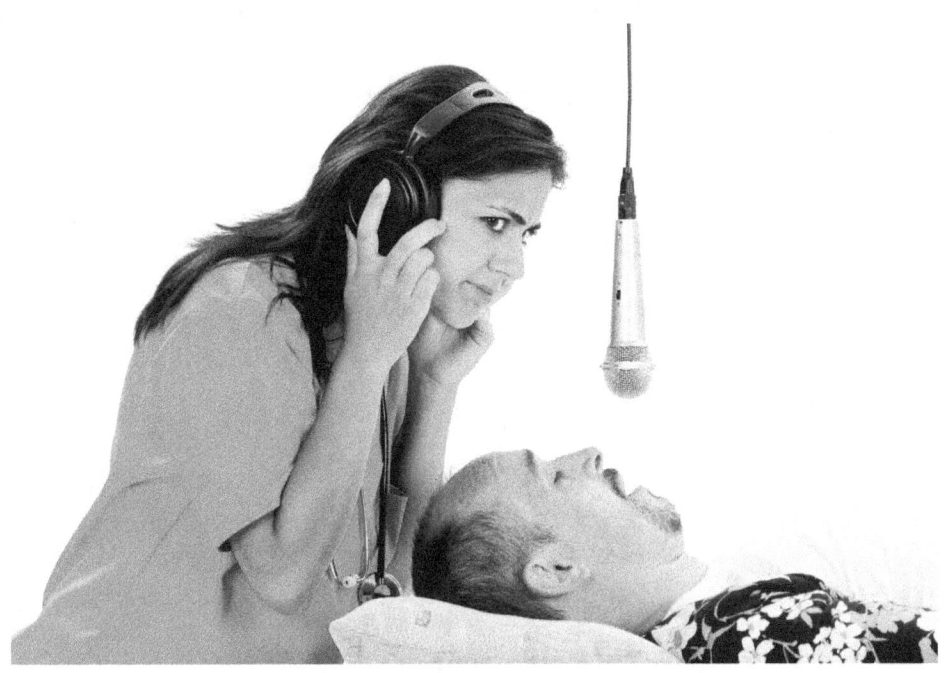

Sleep studies are normally performed in a sleep center or a sleep lab. This may or may not be in a hospital. If the study is conducted in the sleep center, you may have an overnight stay. However, this is not always etched in stone.

The good thing about sleep studies is you will not endure any pain. The only thing that may affect you is skin irritation from the sensors. When the sensors are removed from your skin, you will not experience any more irritation.

If your sleep study is during the day, bring a book or a magazine to keep you from getting bored. Although the risks of sleep studies are minimal, these studies take time (at least several hours). There are different tests for sleep studies. One of them is called a polysomnogram (poly-SOM-no-gram) or PSG test. This test is conducted in a sleep center or sleep lab. More than likely with this test, it will require an overnight stay.

You will have electrodes and monitors on your scalp, face, chest, limbs and fingers. As you are sleeping, the following items will be monitored:

- The movement of your eyes
- The activity in your brain
- The activity in your muscles
- The rate of your heart
- The rhythm of your heart
- Blood pressure
- Air movement in and out of your lungs
- How much oxygen is in your blood

As you sleep, the staff on duty will use sensors to check on your as you sleep during the night. After the PSG is complete, the sleep specialist will go over the results with you. They will be able to determine whether or not you have sleep apnea and if it is serious or not. From the results, they will be able to chart a course of treatment.

A Multiple Sleep Latency Test or MSLT, is used to determine how sleepy you are in the daytime. This test is usually performed after a PSG. You will have devices placed on your scalp for monitoring purposes.

With this test, you will have to take a nap at least five times at twenty minutes for each one. This is supposed to be done every two hours during times that you would be alert. The testers will check how long it will take you to go to sleep and how long you napped.

For those people who take less than five minutes to get to sleep are more likely candidates for a sleep disorder. When the testing is completed, the sleep specialist will provide you with the results and consult you about treatment options.

Where To Find A Sleep Specialist

If you need assistance finding a sleep specialist, there are several organizations that can assist you with that, such as:

- American Academy of Sleep Medicine (AASM)
- American Board of Sleep Medicine (ABSM)
- American Academy of Dental Sleep Medicine (AADSM)

These organizations are made up of physicians, researchers and dentists that work with people affected with this sleep disorder. They work to further the advancement of sleep medicine and sleep research.

The physicians and researches that serve on the related boards are noted as "Board Certified" in the specialty of sleep medicine. The ABSM keeps an updated listing of sleep specialists. They can be located by state or by their name. The AADSM keeps and updated listing of dentists that specialize in treating sleep apnea patients by using oral devices.

CHAPTER 6: SLEEP APNEA SYMPTOMS IN CHILDREN

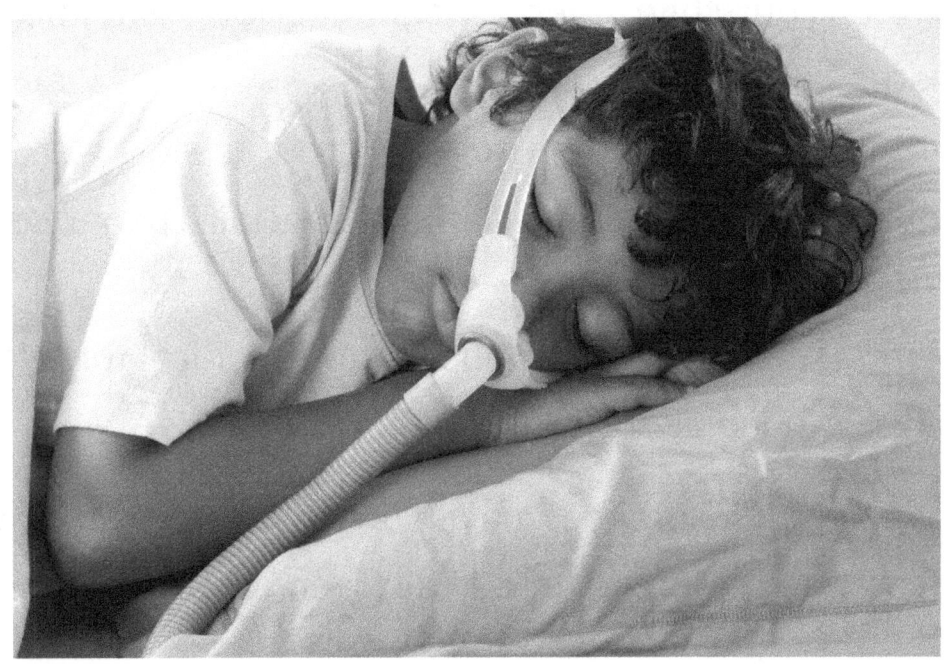

Children who are diagnosed with sleep apnea can be hyperactive and aggressive. They can also suffer greatly in their studies. Sometimes they may sleep different than normal. They may also wet the bed. During the daytime hours, some of them will breathe through their mouth instead of breathing through their nose.

Snoring loudly, snorting, gasping for air and temporary stoppage in breathing all are signs of sleep apnea. Basically, their signs and symptoms are parallel with what adults have.

Even with this, physicians cannot always detect this sleep disorder in children. They figure because most are hyperactive anyway, that it's not a big deal.

There are some things that you can do to find out if your child actually has sleep apnea:

- Check with your child's pediatrician and let them know what's going on.
- Consult with an ENT (ear, nose and throat) specialist.
- Consult with a pulmonologist (lung specialist) that specializes in children.
- Psychiatrists, psychologists and other medical providers can also help with a diagnosis.

If you have health insurance, make sure to consult with them first to see if you need referrals for certain medical providers.

If there is further testing to be done, check to see if the physicians are board certified to treat children with sleep apnea. Don't be afraid to ask for their credentials. Besides, this is your child's health that you're dealing with. With them, any diagnosis can require delicate care and attentiveness.

The physician will also need to find out if they are taking medications and if the child is allergic to anything. Also, advise them of any issues with their behavior and development. In addition to that, provide them with information on their nightly sleep patterns and if they take naps.

The child may have to take a sleep study or polysomnogram (PSG) to determine the severity of their sleep apnea. There are other tests that are given to make a determination. They include:

- An electroencephalogram (EEG), which is use to measure the waves of the brain;
- An electroculogram (EOG), which is used for chin and eye measurements;
- Both of these tests are used to check on the different sleep stages;
- An electrocardiogram (EKG), which is used for rhythm and heart rate measurements;
- Tests using chest bands for breathing movement measurements;
- Tests using more monitors for levels of oxygen and levels carbon dioxide in the child's blood.

The majority of the sleep studies for children require an overnight stay. There are not a lot of medical facilities that specialize in sleep apnea for children. Even with that, the ones that are used for adults will utilize them to test children as well.

Check the facility to find out if they work with children that may have this sleep disorder. As with adults, check various organizations and groups to find a qualified sleep specialist.

Also, as with adults, if sleep apnea goes untreated in children, they can also experience serious health issues down the road. Children can also get worse with their behavioral patterns and academics in school if they are not treated in a timely manner. Don't take for granted that they may just be going through a difficult time when it could very well be sleep apnea.

CHAPTER 7: TREATING SLEEP APNEA

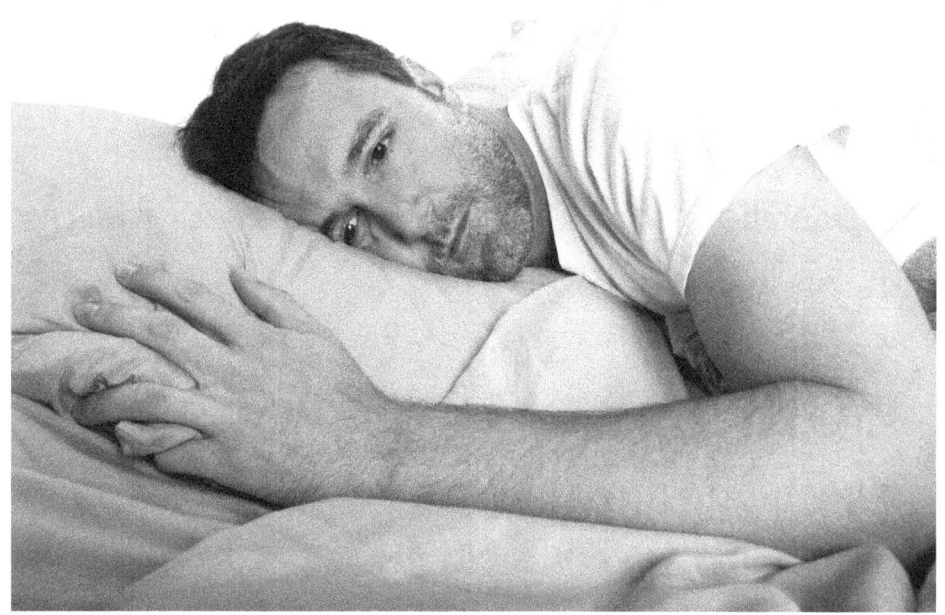

The purpose of treating sleep apnea (obstructive) is to allow the patient to be able to breathe regularly as they sleep. The treatment also helps to get relief from snoring loudly and being chronically sleepy during the day.

Treatment of sleep apnea also helps to reduce medical problems, such as heart disease, diabetes, high blood pressure and other medical conditions.

Types of Treatments

There are different types of treatments to use for sleep apnea. Here are some of the more common ones:

- Lifestyle changes
- CPAP

- Mouthpiece or oral appliance
- Surgery
- Therapies

With treatment, you can get more sleep and get rid of being tired and sleepy during the daytime. Your overall health will improve along with you being happier that you are able to get more sleep without being interrupted at night.

It can also help your mate get more sleep as well. You won't be disturbing them by getting up at different times of the night making snorting and gasping noises.

Chapter 8: Making Lifestyle Changes

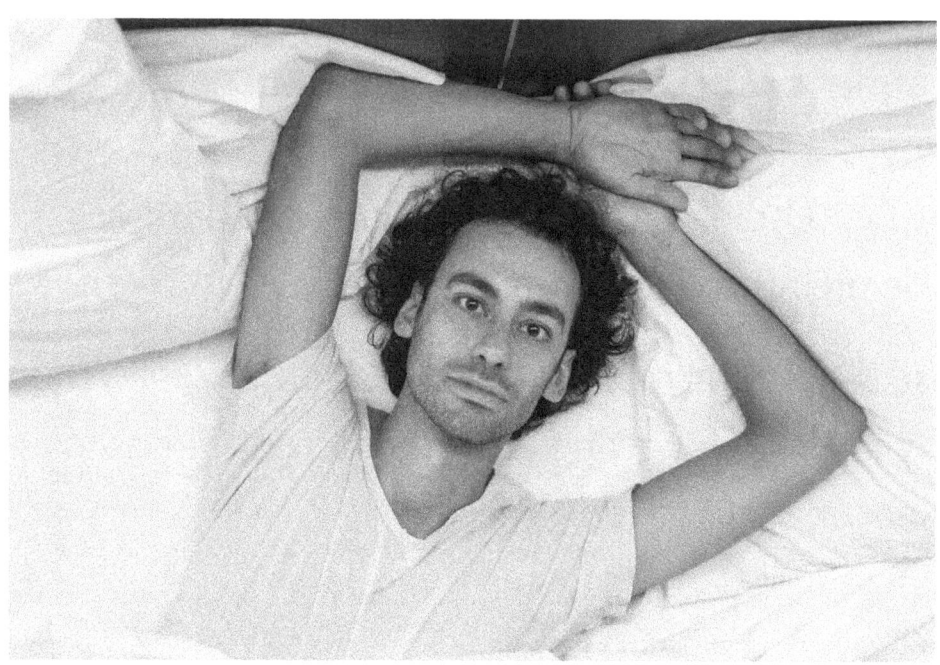

If you sleep on your back, you are more apt to develop sleep apnea. The way you position yourself as you lie down on the bed can make or break you. It can determine how many times you experience obstructive sleep apnea. It also determines how mild or severe the sleep apnea can affect you.

Sometimes it has to do with gravity. Gravity can cause your throat not to get enough air when you are lying on your back. For those who sleep on their back can experience up to eighty apneas per hour. They can get rid of this dilemma is they change and sleep on either their left or right side. However, if you are overweight or obese, this may not help much.

You can make some lifestyle changes in order to deal with obstructive sleep apnea and central sleep apnea:

- If you are overweight or obese, losing weight can help. Weight loss can help your throat to be less restrictive. Eat more healthy fruits and vegetables. Be more physically active. If you are not sure how to go about losing weight, consult with your physician.
- Leave the sleeping pills and related medicines alone. Also, don't drink alcohol as a sedative to get you to sleep.
- The passageway of your nasal area should not be blocked. If you have trouble keeping them open, use a nasal spray or stick. You can also use decongestants, but it's not for long-term use.
- If you are used to sleeping on your back, that can pose a problem. Try sleeping on your side or your stomach. If you sleep on your back, your tongue and soft palate of your throat will sit on the back. This creates a blockage of the throat's airway.
- Elevate the head of your bed to improve your level of oxygen that you're taking in.
- If you smoke cigarettes, you need to kick the habit as soon as possible.

Alternative treatments, such as acupuncture have been used to treat sleep apnea, but there is more research to be done. Because of this, do not use this method as a means to get rid of this condition. Consult with your physician before considering any alternative treatment for sleep apnea.

Chapter 9: Other Treatments for Sleep Apnea

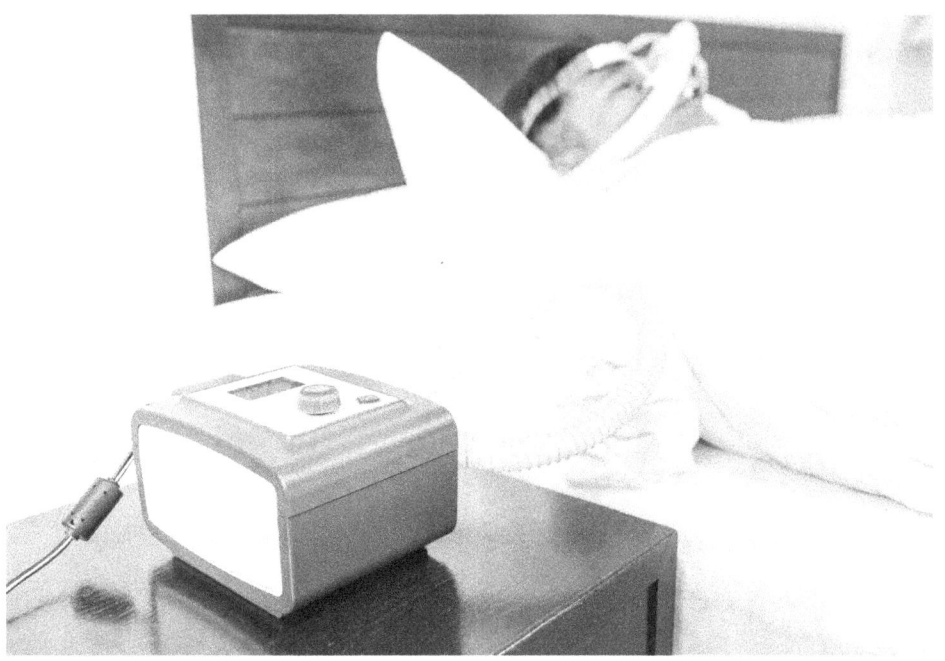

If lifestyle changes don't help to treat your sleep apnea, then your case is more severe than what you first thought. Here are some other treatments that may help:

CPAP (Continuous Positive Airway Pressure)

CPAP (Continuous Positive Airway Pressure) is a method where a machine produces air pressure. In order to receive it, you have to wear a mask. The mask is situated on your nose while you're sleeping.

When you are using CPAP, you receive more air pressure than you would if you were just breathing in air from the outside. The air pressure with this machine helps to keep the passageways of your upper airway open. This helps to prevent snoring and apnea.

In the beginning, not everyone that uses this machine will feel comfortable with it. Because of the way it's made, it may not feel uncomfortable. However, with adjustments and making the straps fit properly, you will be able to get used to wearing it.

However, if the mask you have is not settling in, then you may have to find another one. In addition to that, you can use a humidifier along with the CPAP for additional comfort.

There may be times when you have other problems. However, don't stop using it. Instead, check with your physician to see what can be done and make additional corrections or adjustments. If you have gained weight, the settings for the air pressure any have to be changed.

Possible Side Effects With CPAP

During the first few nights that you wear this device, it can get on your nerves because it is not automatically comfortable to wear. It makes you want to stop the treatment for sleep apnea. However, it would defeat the purpose. What you can do is use the device with low air pressure starting out.

Most people that use CPAP say that they experience side effects. Most of them are dealing with the mask itself. You can select a mask that provides comfort and prevents it from leaking a lot of air pressure.

Here are some of the side effects that you may experience with the device:

- Irritated eyes.
- More air pressure than usual—you can have a difficult time exhaling when that happens.
- Experience infections in the upper respiratory area if you don't keep the device clean.
- Nose and throat irritation.
- Dry mouth.
- Sore mouth.
- Congestion in the nasal area.
- Nose sores from wearing the device too tight.
- Discomfort of the chest muscles

There will be times when the CPAP will have to be adjusted. Your physician or a sleep specialist can teach you how to do this. Once you learn how to do it, you will be able to save money by not having to make visits to see your physician or specialist (unless absolutely necessary).

You can also get devices that will help you to get more air in your throat. They are adjustable and made to fit your needs in order to get more air flowing through your throat. The device adjusts the air pressure while you're sleeping. You don't have to push a button or use a dial to adjust it. The adjustment is done automatically as you sleep.

A mouthpiece or an oral appliance is another option if the CPAP doesn't work out for you. This device is used to keep your throat open so that you can get air. It can help those who are dealing with mild sleep apnea.

Even though the CPAP is more effective than the mouthpiece, the latter has been proven easier for some people to use while they're sleeping. It opens your throat by moving your lower jaw forward. Doing this can help your snoring and treat the mild obstructive sleep apnea.

You can get a mouthpiece from a dentist. It may take a few attempts to find the right one that you are comfortable with. It's important that you check with the dentist every six months after you start wearing it.

After the first year of wear, check in with the dentist once a year. You want to make sure that it is still fitting right and working properly. If you are feeling any discomfort, don't hesitate to contact the dentist for a possible adjustment.

Surgery

Surgery is another option to use in order to treat sleep apnea. With the surgical procedure, excess tissue is removed from your nose or your throat. This procedure is only performed in a hospital.

Another option is to shrink or stiffen the excess tissue or the lower jaw can be reset. When the tissue is being shrunk or stiffened, the procedure is usually performed in a doctor's office or it can be performed in a hospital.

If the shrinking procedure is performed, you may have to get some shots in the tissue area. If the excess tissue needs to be shrunk more, you may need other treatments besides the shots. Also, the stiffening process includes the physician creating a small cut in the excess tissue and placing a small piece of plastic which is stiff.

During the pre-surgery, you will be administered some medicine that is to make you go to sleep. So, during the surgery, you will be out and not feel anything until you wake up. When the surgery is performed in the hospital, you may experience pain in your throat for approximately seven to fourteen days afterwards.

Here are some surgical options to treat sleep apnea and help you rest better:

UPPP (Uvulopalatopharyngoplasty) - This is a procedure where tissue is taken from the back of your mouth. Tissue is also removed from the top portion of your throat. In addition to removing tissue, your tonsils and adenoids are also removed.

With this surgery, your snoring may stop; however, since there is still tissue further down in your throat, it is unlikely that it will treat or cure your sleep apnea. With the tissue remaining there, your air passage is not open. With UPPP surgery, you will have to go to a hospital to have the surgery.

With this surgery, you will experience a lot of pain. You will be recovering for several weeks. This surgery is only performed on people who are experiencing severe obstructive sleep apnea. Even then, there are only some who undergo this procedure.

This is not one of those surgeries where you can get up and it's back to business as usual. If you're able to have the UPPP surgery, you may risk having some complications, including:

- The soft palate and throat muscles may not work properly.
- Your throat may get infected if no antibiotics are given prior to the surgery.
- You may have problems swallowing.
- You may experience fluids coming up through your mouth or your nose.
- You may not be able to smell.

Having surgery to help you sleep better is not a guarantee. You may still have a recurrence of sleep apnea episodes. Even using CPAP will not be as effective after the surgery. There are some oral surgeries that can be performed:

Tracheostomy – This surgery is performed if previous treatments did not help you. It is also used if your sleep apnea is severe to the point where it's a matter of life of death.

From an opening in your neck, a tube made of metal or plastic is inserted and used for you to breathe from. The opening stays covered in the daytime and uncovered at night. You need air to come in and out of your lungs as you sleep.

Maxillomandibular advancement – This surgical procedure is used to prevent obstruction of your throat by making the space larger where your tongue and soft palate is situated.

The upper and lower portion of your jaw is moved toward the front. This is how the enlargement is created. This procedure is complex, that it may take an oral surgeon and orthodontist to perform it together.

Surgeons use lasers to get rid of unnecessary tissues in the back of your throat. They can also use radiofrequency energy. Both of these procedures are good to use for treating snoring. Even though they can be use to relieve snoring, they should not be used to treat obstructive sleep apnea.

There are additional procedures that are used to relieve snoring. Some of them can help with treating sleep apnea. However, the procedures are not cures for this sleep disorder.

They include:

- Getting rid of enlarged tonsils or adenoids
- Nasal surgery – polyps are removed or a partition positioned between your nostrils is straightened out.

Additional surgical procedures that are used may deal with abnormalities on your face. There are also surgical procedures that deal with additional obstructions. Both of these can cause you to have sleep apnea. The procedures can be performed together or solo.

Other surgeries include:

- Plastic surgery on the chin
- Tongue advancement – this procedure involves a cut at the intersection of the jawbone and the tongue.
- Hyoid surgery – the bone under the chin that can move is moved toward the front. As it moves, the muscle of the tongue moves with it.

Having surgery to treat apnea is not a guarantee. If depends on what kind of surgery it is and the details of the sleep apnea.

For central and complex sleep apnea, different therapies can be used. Some of them include:

- CPAP (Continuous Positive Airway Pressure)
- Medical treatments for heart, neuromuscular issues
- BiPAP (Bilevel Positive Airway Pressure) – this is when higher pressure is used for inhaling. When you exhale, the air pressure gets lower. This helps to strengthen your breathing pattern if you have central sleep apnea. The device can be set to automatic mode if it detects that you haven't breathed into it after a few seconds.
- ASV (Adaptive servo-ventilation) – This is a new airflow device that gets a feel for how you breathe normally. It keeps your breathing pattern information in a computer.

While you're sleeping, the ASV works to keep your breathing pattern at a normal rate and get rid of any breathing pauses. If you have central sleep apnea, this method may work better for you than CPAP.

Sleep Apnea Pillows

There are some people who do get the recommended amount of sleep, but still get up fatigued. This can be related to their snoring. Snoring is a very serious medical issue. To combat that, sleep apnea pillows can be used.

Sleep apnea pillows have been known to treat sleep apnea in some people. Before you try one, you must know whether or not you are just snoring or if the snoring is a result of sleep apnea (obstructive). However, even it is snoring without the condition, you can still use one of these pillows to reduce your snoring, if nothing else.

Sleep apnea pillows can help the airway of your throat stay open. Because sleep apnea causes your breathing to be irregular and interrupted, the pillow works to make your breathing regular again. The irregular and interrupted breathing usually happens during the evening when you are sleeping.

The special pillows are designed with panels of foam that are elevated, unlike a regular pillow. The elevation works to keep your head slanted. This helps to increase your breathing pattern to make it regular and uninterrupted again.

Sleep apnea pillows can be made to where they can be used in more than one sleeping position. They are adjustable, so that you can sleep in the way that is most comfortable for you. They provide you with plenty of support so that you can get a good night's sleep.

The sleep apnea pillow also helps in the following ways in regard to sleep apnea:

- Blocked airways are opened—this helps with snoring relief and sleep apnea
- Provides comfort and support so that you can get a good night's sleep
- Relieves you from the fatigue that you experience as a result of your sleep apnea condition
- The pillow allows you to sleep like a baby

There are people who are chronic snorers that have never used these types of pillows and don't want to try them. They would rather get sleeping pills and end up getting dependent on them. Medication is not a good alternative to assist you with your snoring or sleep apnea. In fact, medication is not recommended because it has proven not to be effective.

CHAPTER 10: IMPORTANT FACTS ABOUT SLEEP APNEA

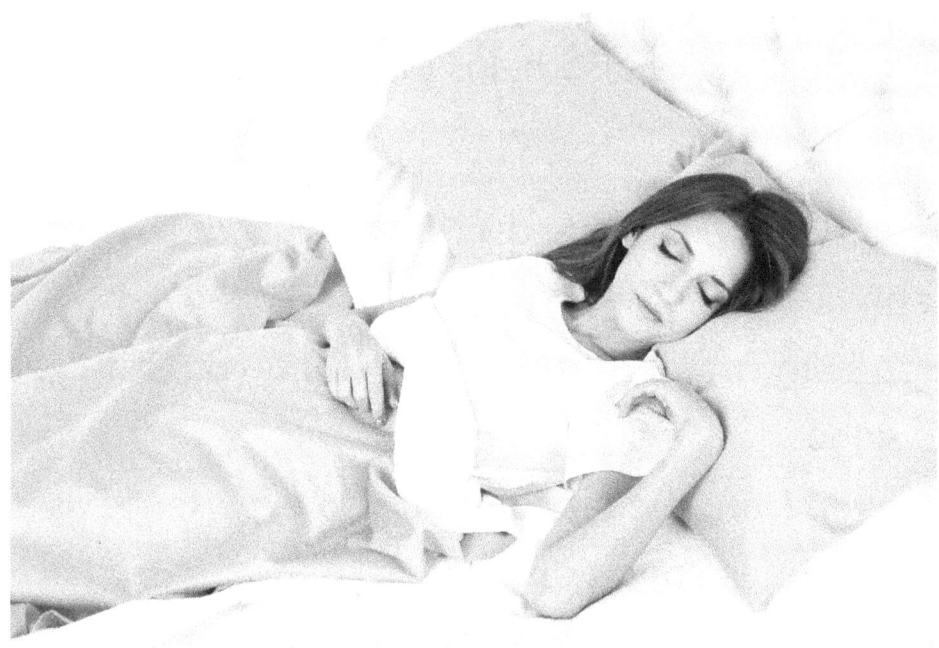

Here are some important points that you should know about sleep apnea:

- Sleep apnea is a chronic condition in which your sleep is interrupted more than three nights every week.
- Because snoring is normal for some people, this sleep disorder can be easily undetected.
- Obstructive sleep apnea is the most common of the three that are mentioned.
- Being chronically sleepy in the daytime can cause you to have a work-related accident or injury.
- If you are overweight or obese and suffering from sleep apnea, work on getting your weight down. Once you do, don't put the pounds back on.

- A family member can determine something may be wrong when the person is choking and gasping for air and not getting enough sleep.
- There are different ways to get treated for sleep apnea. Depending on the severity of your condition, the physician and sleep specialist will work to get the best treatment for you.
- People should not make fun of those who are suffering from sleep apnea. This is a very serious sleep disorder that should be treated with urgency.
- Children that have behavioral problems and issues with academics are often overlooked. These signs are usually not associated with sleep apnea.

Chapter 11: Conclusion

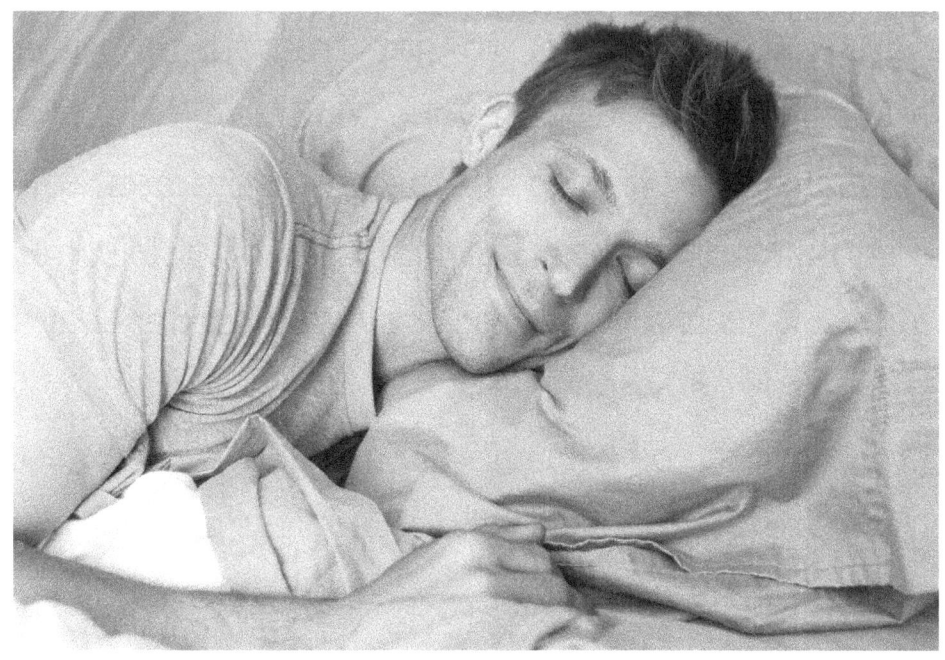

With sleep apnea, it is a condition where the symptoms are not easily recognized. However, down the road, someone may notice something. Keep in mind that just because your snoring may be chronic, it's not a guarantee that you have the sleep disorder. The only way that you'll find out is through exams and sleep studies.

It's important that if you or someone suspects something different in your sleeping pattern, that you consult a physician as soon as possible. It could mean the difference of getting treatment in time to prevent serious health issues.

Meet the Author

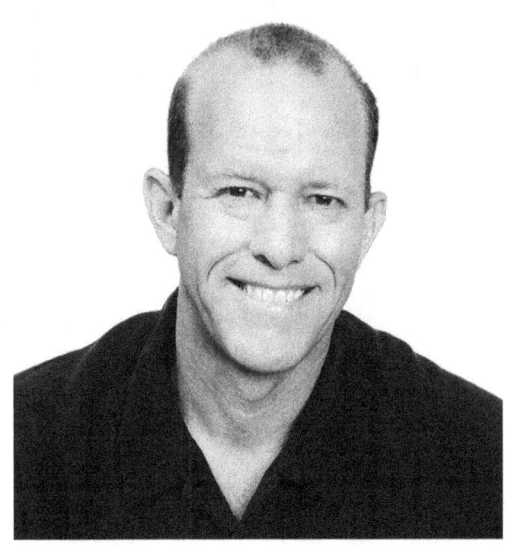

Hayden Anderson has a passion for helping others obtain peace and wellness. Sometimes that means changing lifestyle habits and addressing medical complexities through nutrition and alternative medicine. Hayden has years of experience in the area of holistic health, yoga, and meditation. He uses his experience and knowledge to change people's perception of eastern medicine.

As a kid Hayden suffered from a chronic illness that doctor's treated with medication. Hayden's parents were satisfied with doctor's maintaining his condition but Hayden wanted more. At nineteen Hayden became obsessed with eastern medicine and took control of his health. Through the use of herbs and dietary changes to complement his blood type, he was able throw away prescription medication that he had taken daily for as long as he could remember. He never looked back and is passionate about sharing his knowledge with others.

Hayden, his wife and kids enjoy spending time outdoors, growing their own food and herbs, sharing their day with each other around the family dinner table and game nights with old fashioned board games like Parcheesi, Aggravation, Sorry, Clue and Life.

More Books by Hayden Anderson

Irritable Bowel Syndrome: IBS Symptoms, Remedies and Prevention

Toothache Relief Naturally: Home Remedies to Eliminate and Prevent Tooth Pain

www.ingramcontent.com/pod-product-compliance
Lightning Source LLC
LaVergne TN
LVHW081546060526
838200LV00048B/2232